BRAIN GAMES TO EXERCISE YOUR MIND

Protect Your Brain from Memory Loss and Other Age-Related Disorders

GARY SMALL, M.D.
and GIGI VORGAN

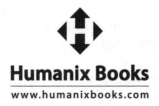

Humanix Books
www.humanixbooks.com

Humanix Books

BRAIN GAMES TO EXERCISE YOUR MIND
Copyright © 2023 by Humanix Books
All rights reserved

Humanix Books, P.O. Box 20989, West Palm Beach, FL 33416, USA
www.humanixbooks.com | info@humanixbooks.com

Humanix Books is a division of Humanix Publishing, LLC. Its trademark, consisting of the words "Humanix Books," is registered in the
Patent and Trademark Office and in other countries.

Disclaimer: The information presented in this book is not specific
medical advice for any individual and should not substitute medical
advice from a health professional. If you have (or think you may have)
a medical problem, speak to your doctor or a health professional
immediately about your risk and possible treatments. Do not engage
in any care or treatment without consulting a medical professional.

Portions of this work have previously appeared in *2 Weeks to a
Younger Brain* and *The Small Guide to Alzheimer's Disease*, published by Humanix Books.

ISBN: 9-781-63006-189-0 (Paperback)
ISBN: 9-781-63006-190-6 (E-book)

Printed in the United States of America
10 9 8 7 6 5 4 3 2 1

"As you get older three things happen. The first is your memory goes, and I can't remember the other two."

—SIR NORMAN WISDOM

CONTENTS

INTRODUCTION

Most people know that if they engage in regular exercise, their muscles will grow and get stronger. If they commit to an aerobic conditioning routine, their heart health will improve, and they will live longer. But many people don't realize that exercising their minds actually builds brain muscle and helps protect against the decline that often comes with aging.

Accumulating scientific evidence supports the idea that brain workouts—doing puzzles, taking classes, playing games, reading books, or even engaging in stimulating conversations—can lower a person's risk for age-related cognitive decline. Initial studies supporting this notion included a large epidemiological sample of people in the community in order to determine if people who attended college experienced lower rates of future cognitive decline and dementia, which is defined as a cognitive impairment severe enough to interfere with a person's independence.

Several years ago, investigators from the Karolinska Institute in Sweden, the University of Cambridge in the UK, and other European research centers reviewed the educational histories of over seventeen thousand patients with a diagnosis of Alzheimer's dementia and compared them to those of thirty-seven thousand cognitively healthy control subjects without dementia. The research team concluded that higher educational attainment is associated with a reduced risk of getting Alzheimer's disease. The research team estimated that for each year of educational achievement, the risk of developing Alzheimer's disease was reduced by about 10 percent.

Although those are fairly impressive odds, they still don't definitively prove that the mental stimulation associated with pursuing a college degree actually protects the brain. Another explanation could be that people with increased formal education are more aware that healthy lifestyle habits—like not smoking, getting regular physical exercise, and staying on top of personal medical needs—will protect their brain health.

Other research findings add support to the idea that the old adage "use it or lose it" may apply to the brain as well as the body. A study of more than three hundred cognitively normal middle-aged adults enrolled in the Wisconsin Registry for Alzheimer's Prevention indicated that research volunteers who engaged in more frequent and extensive cognitive activity, including game playing, had larger brain volumes in regions controlling memory and thinking. These volunteers also scored higher on tests of memory, language, and other cognitive skills.

In my own research, I hypothesized that it is possible to observe heightened neural activity in the brain when people engage in cognitively stimulating activities. To test this hypothesis, my research team assessed patterns of brain neural activation in cognitively normal middle-aged and older adults while they performed a simulated online search task during functional magnetic resonance imaging (MRI) scanning. We found that volunteers with prior internet-search experience showed a more than twofold increase in the extent of neural activation compared to those who had never searched online before. We then trained the internet-naïve volunteers on the basics of searching online and instructed them to practice internet searching for one hour each day for a week. We repeated the functional MRI scans while these internet-trained volunteers performed the simulated search and found significant increases in neural activity compared with their baseline scans, particularly in the frontal lobe of the brain, the area that controls reasoning and decision-making.

Additional research has shown that computer apps and video games can train our brains and improve our problem-solving capabilities, help us focus attention, and shorten our reaction time. Some studies have even shown that certain video games can train working memory and boost problem-solving skills. Working memory, a form of short-term memory, is what temporarily holds information in the mind long enough to use it, such as hearing a phone number and then dialing it right away. The research indicates that when you train your working memory, it can translate into an improvement in fluid intelligence—the capacity to think logically and solve problems.

Even though it is difficult to definitively prove that playing games and solving riddles will fortify brain health, brainteasers and puzzles still provide an opportunity for mental fun. The key is to train but not strain the brain, which means it is best to find puzzles that are challenging but not overly difficult. If your brain games are too easy, you'll get bored, but if they are too difficult, they may be stressful and cause you to give up on them.

We have lots of options for stimulating our minds, ranging from game playing and socializing to traveling, taking classes, learning languages, or completing crosswords or Sudoku puzzles. A helpful strategy is to find stimulating activities that you enjoy and try to "cross-train" your brain. That means alternating a visual-spatial puzzle like a jigsaw with a language puzzle like a word scramble. Cross-training the brain adds variety, which keeps our minds interested in the mental activity longer.

Scientists at the University of California, San Francisco, performed research on a video game that required players to steer an animated race car along a winding road while informative and distracting street signs pop up. The researchers found that older adults who played the game for a month experienced improved multitasking skills to the point that they performed at the same level as untrained twenty-year-olds. Other studies have shown that surgeons who play video games make fewer errors in the operating room. It is likely that action games that train attention and reaction time also improve surgical skills, so playing certain video games can be a form of mental exercise that provides practical benefits, whether it's performing surgery or piloting an airplane.

A form of mental exercise that offers additional practical benefits for middle-aged and older adults involves learning and using memory methods that compensate for everyday forgetfulness. Most memory techniques include three important tasks: focusing attention, visualizing the information that you want to remember, and creating mental associations that link those visual images, making them easier to recall.

The most frequent reason that people are forgetful is that they are not paying attention in the first place. Doing exercises that help focus attention is a great way to start to strengthen your memory skills. Creating mental images of what you want to remember will leverage your brain's inborn visual abilities, and creating meaningful associations will make the information more memorable. These methods can be used to recall names and faces and items on a to-do list, as well as help you find those keys, glasses, and other items that most people commonly misplace.

Keeping our brains healthy and our minds sharp involves more than just mental exercise. Considerable research points to a formula for successful brain aging that incorporates mental exercise along with physical workouts, healthy nutrition, stress management, and social engagement. Each of these lifestyle habits contributes to brain health in a variety of ways.

When it comes to physical exercise, you don't have to become a triathlete to keep your brain healthy. Prior research suggests that a twenty-minute brisk walk each day may lower your risk for dementia. That rapid walk may also lift your mood because it causes your body to produce endorphins, which are natural antidepressants. Workouts also produce brain-derived neurotrophic factor (BDNF), a protein that gets your brain cells to sprout new branches and communicate more effectively.

Investigators at the University of Illinois have demonstrated that regular aerobic conditioning can increase the size of the brain's memory-forming region and improve attention and reasoning abilities. After six months of regular cardiovascular conditioning, middle-aged and older volunteers were shown to have larger hippocampal memory centers compared to a control group that only did stretching without walking. Hippocampal size increased even more for volunteers who continued their walking routine for an entire year.

Social engagement bolsters brain health in several ways. Dr. Oscar Ybarra and his colleagues studied cognitive abilities after a stimulating discussion and found that a ten-minute conversation results in significantly better memory performance and an improved speed of mental processing compared to watching a sitcom rerun. Conversations are like mental calisthenics that bolster neuronal networks. By engaging in daily discussions on topics of interest, you keep your neural circuits strong. And conversing with an empathic friend may help lower your stress levels, which can further bolster your brain health.

Learning other ways to effectively manage stress will improve brain health by reducing cortisol levels. This stress hormone has been shown to cause temporary memory impairment after being injected into healthy volunteers. The good news is that such impairment is passing: meditation and other relaxation techniques not only improve mood but also boost cognitive abilities.

Healthy nutrition can protect brain health too. Heightened brain inflammation that accumulates with age can accelerate cognitive decline. However, ingesting omega-3 fatty acids, which are found in fish and nuts, helps lower this inflammation. Fresh fruits and vegetables contain antioxidants that can protect brain cells from wear and tear due to age-related oxidative stress. Diabetes can double the risk of getting dementia, and avoiding processed foods and refined sugars will lower a person's risk for diabetes.

The brain games in this book are an excellent start to help you create your own regular routine of mental aerobics. For example, in my house, we like to start each morning with a stimulating conversation about the day's news and then knock off a Sudoku puzzle. The conversation exercises brain regions throughout the cortex (outer region) that control language and reasoning. The Sudoku puzzle activates the left hemisphere (mathematical skills) and right hemisphere (visual-spatial abilities). If we have time after that, we'll try a crossword, which tweaks brain areas controlling visual-spatial abilities and language skills. Add a healthy breakfast following a good night's sleep, and you are on your way to a brain-healthy day.

How much mental stimulation should you engage in each day? That will depend on your lifestyle. If you have an extremely challenging job that requires effortful mental work throughout the day, you may prefer brain games that are more relaxing and not concern yourself so much with building brain muscle. If your job is more mundane and less mentally challenging, you may wish to push harder on your brain games. The scientific evidence is clear that these nongenetic lifestyle factors have a significant impact on brain health as we age. And whatever mental exercise routine you adopt, try to make it a habit. For healthy lifestyle choices to have an effect, we need to engage in them on a regular basis for the long haul.

Remember, our minds crave variety, so be sure to change things up if you find that your brain games routine is becoming too rote. Keep challenging yourself to achieve more to further expand your mental horizons. And most of all, have fun with your mental exercise as you strengthen your memory and fortify your brain cells.

Gary Small, M.D.
Gigi Vorgan

PART 1:

BRAIN GAMES

GETTING STARTED

KNOW WHICH MENTAL SKILLS YOU ARE TRAINING

- **Visual-spatial:** Mazes, jigsaw puzzles, action video games
- **Language:** Crosswords, Scrabble, letter scramble games
- **Problem-solving:** Chess, number games like KenKen or Sudoku, riddles and logic games
- **Memory and concentration:** Match games, card games like gin or fish, Trivial Pursuit

OPTIMIZING YOUR BRAIN GAME EXPERIENCE

- Brain exercises should be challenging and fun to keep you playing for the long haul.
- If a game is too hard, dial it back to an easier level.
- If a game becomes too easy, increase to the next level of difficulty or switch to another game.

- Search the internet to exercise your neural circuits.
- Your brain likes variety, so vary your mental workouts to bolster both sides of your brain and diverse regions.
- Try games that enhance specific mental abilities, including multitasking and fluid intelligence.
- HAVE FUN.

HOW TO USE THIS BOOK

Dr. Small's games and puzzles are short, single-page brain teasers that will exercise your mind but not break it.

The puzzles should not take long to solve. But take all the time you need.

And feel free to skip a tough one and go back to it later—it might be much easier after you take a break.

Tackle a couple a day or all in one go. Then go back and try them again, giving yourself more time or challenge yourself with less time.

The solution to each brain game can be found on the following page, so make sure you do not flip the page until you are ready to see the solution. And then, when you are ready, move on to the next brain teaser.

DON'T GIVE UP exercising your mind.

HAVE FUN improving your memory.

ENJOY—BETTER BRAIN HEALTH.

BRAIN GAME #1

Getting Started with an Easy Brain Teaser

Here's a "beginner" brain teaser from Dr. Small to get started.

Dr. Small is confident that your brain can unscramble the following sentence quickly:

Teh rihgt psyichal adn mtneal eerxcsie acn ekep oury bairn oyugn.

Turn the page for the solution. ➤

BRAIN GAME #1 SOLUTION

The right physical and mental exercise can keep your brain young.

BRAIN GAME #2

Numbers Game

This exercise will help you think outside the box and strengthen the right side of your brain that controls visual and spatial abilities.

Take five toothpicks and arrange them to display the number 5, as seen below.

See if you can rearrange them (without bending or breaking them) to display the number 16.

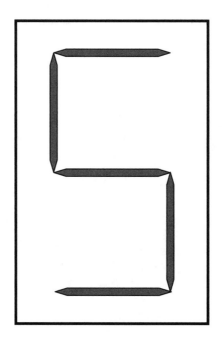

Turn the page for the solution. ➤

BRAIN GAME #2 SOLUTION

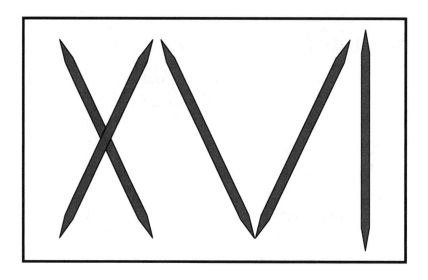

BRAIN GAME #3

Word Chain

This mental workout will strengthen your brain's left hemisphere (or the right hemisphere if you are left-handed).

That is the side of the brain that controls language skills.

Starting with the word TALL, change one letter at a time to a new letter until you have the word RAIN.

Hint: Each change must spell a proper word.

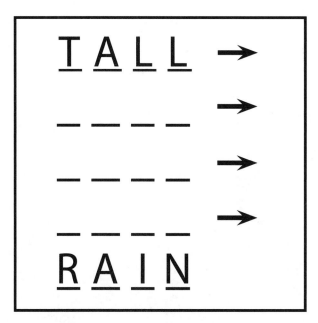

Turn the page for the solution. ⟶

BRAIN GAME #3 SOLUTION

T A L L →

F A L L →

F A I L →

R A I L →

R A I N

BRAIN GAME #4

Boosting Spatial Ability

Boost your right-brain visual and spatial abilities by quickly counting the number of squares in the figure below.

How many do you see?

Hint: Be sure to count the squares within the squares.

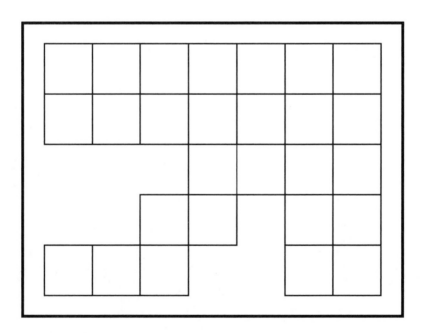

Turn the page for the solution. ➤

BRAIN GAME #4 SOLUTION

Thirty-two squares

BRAIN GAME #5

Name That Color

Here's a brain teaser that will help activate the neural circuits within your brain's left hemisphere.

Rearrange the letters to find the four colors mixed up below.

Hint: Only one is a primary color.

EGERN

GENRAO

TOVEIL

EOLWYL

Turn the page for the solution. ➤

BRAIN GAME #5 SOLUTION

GREEN

ORANGE

VIOLET

YELLOW (primary color)

BRAIN GAME #6

Right-Brain Exercise: Connect the Dots with Straight-Line Drawing

Here's a brain teaser from Dr. Small's book *2 Weeks to a Younger Brain*.

See if you can draw four straight, connected lines that pass through all eight dots below.

Make sure each line touches each dot only once. You should not lift your pencil from the paper while drawing the lines.

Hint: Free yourself up from one of the usual assumptions you use to connect the dots.

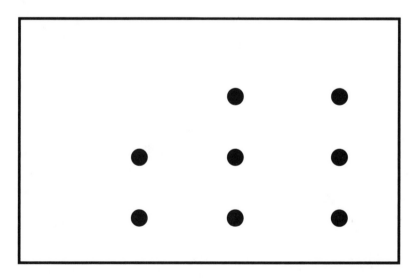

Turn the page for the solution. ➤

BRAIN GAME #6 SOLUTION

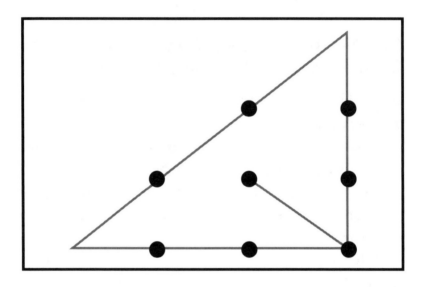

BRAIN GAME #7

The Shopping List

One way to improve your memory is to sort the information you wish to remember into categories.

Here are sixteen items on a shopping list.

First, try to memorize them without changing their order.

Next, sort the items into four categories and try to memorize them again.

It will probably be much easier.

See how many you recall after ten minutes.

Asparagus   Guava   Donuts
Artichokes   Kale   Tomatoes
Ice cream   Egg whites   Fudge
Spinach   Tuna   Grapefruit
Soybeans   Chicken breast
Cookies   Blueberries

Turn the page for the solution. ➤

BRAIN GAME #7 SOLUTION

Vegetables:
Asparagus
Artichokes
Kale
Spinach

Desserts:
Donuts
Ice cream
Cookies
Fudge

Fruits:
Blueberries
Tomatoes
Grapefruit
Guava

Proteins:
Egg whites
Chicken breasts
Soybeans
Tuna

Try this exercise again with less (or more) time—did you do better?

BRAIN GAME #8

Word Fluency: The Ability to Come up with Words

Word fluency is the ability to list items in a particular classification.

Strengthening this mental capacity will fortify the language area of the brain's frontal lobe.

Try this word fluency exercise from Dr. Small's book *2 Weeks to a Younger Brain.*

Set a timer for two minutes and then, using the letters below, jot down as many words as you can containing three or more letters.

Use each letter only once in each word.

Dr. Small was able to come up with seventeen words in two minutes and up to twenty-five words with more time.

How many words can you come up with?

> # E S M T A

Turn the page for the solution. ▶

BRAIN GAME #8 SOLUTION

Here are some of the words you might have come up with:

EAT, EAST, EATS
SAME, SATE, SEAM, SEAT, SMA, STEAM
MAT, MATE, MAST, MATES,
MET, MEAT, MEATS, META
TAM, TAME, TAMES, TASE,
TEA, TEAS, TEAM, TEAMS
ATE

Keep practicing and give yourself more (or less) time.

BRAIN GAME #9

Moving Toothpicks

Let us try a puzzle that will tweak your right brain's visual-spatial circuits.

Below is an array of toothpicks forming six squares.

See if you can remove just three toothpicks so the remaining unmoved toothpicks display two rectangles.

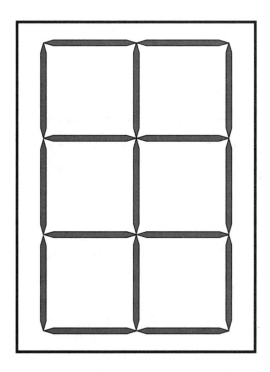

Turn the page for the solution. ──▶

BRAIN GAME #9 SOLUTION

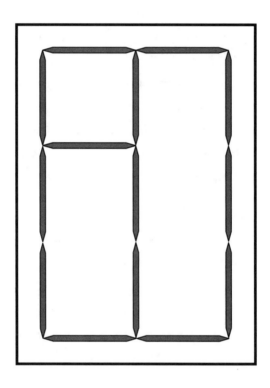

BRAIN GAME #10

Sequencing Numbers

See if you can figure out the next number in this sequence:

1

4

9

16

25

36

___

Turn the page for the solution. ➤

BRAIN GAME #10 SOLUTION

49

The sequence is the square of the numbers:

1

2

3

4

5

6

7

BRAIN GAME #11

Insert Letter

As fast as possible, find one letter to put in front of the following words that will change them into new words.

Hint: The missing letter is the same for each word.

LOW

ROOM

EAST

Turn the page for the solution. ⟶

BRAIN GAME #11 SOLUTION

**Each of the words becomes
a new word if you add the
letter B at the beginning:**

**BLOW
BROOM
BEAST**

How long did it take you?

BRAIN GAME #12

Say What?

Personalized license plates are popular in some parts of the country.

Try to decipher the question posed by the following license plate.

Hint: Think of a fun activity for your body and mind health.

10S NE1

Turn the page for the solution. ➤

BRAIN GAME #12 SOLUTION

Tennis anyone?

BRAIN GAME #13

Find the Letter

Here is a fun left-brain workout.

Try to find the missing letter that completes the word in each of the squares below.

Hint: the missing letter is the same for each word.

D
N
  F
	N T
	   E
	L F

E
D N E
  R
	R R
	 E E
	  I Q

Turn the page for the solution. ➤

BRAIN GAME #13 SOLUTION

The letter is U.

Words:
FUND
FLUENT
REQUIRE
ENDURE

BRAIN GAME #14

Which Is Different?

Assess your visual and spatial skills.

Figure out which object below differs from the others.

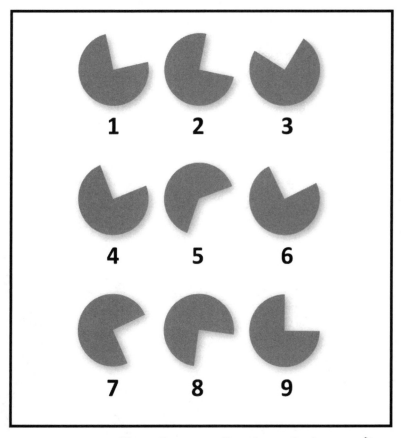

Turn the page for the solution. ➔

BRAIN GAME #14 SOLUTION

Number "5" is different!

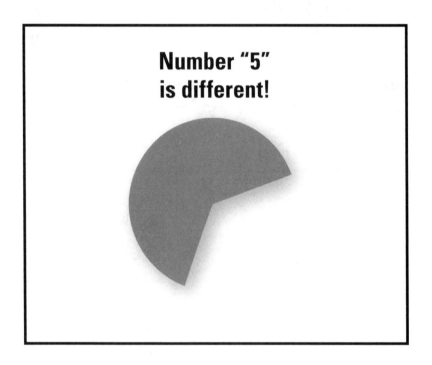

BRAIN GAME #15

Mind (Un)Scramble

See how quickly you can mentally unscramble the letters and make sense of this sentence:

> **The hmuan mnid has phoenmneal pweor.
> Aoccdrnig to rseearchers, the odrer fo ltteer pmacenlet in a wrod deosn't mttaer as lnog as the frist and lsat letetrs are in the corerct pclae.**

Turn the page for the solution. ➤

BRAIN GAME #15 SOLUTION

The human mind has
phenomenal power.
According to researchers, the order
of letter placement in a word doesn't
matter as long as the first and last
letters are in the correct place.

BRAIN GAME #16

Name That Saying

The vowels have been omitted, and the spacing between words has been changed in the following sentence.

Put your brain power to work and see if you can still recognize the proverb:

RL LNG STNG THRS NM SS

Turn the page for the solution. ➤

BRAIN GAME #16 SOLUTION

A ROLLING STONE
GATHERS NO MOSS.

BRAIN GAME #17

Word Chain: Exercise Your Neural Circuits

Have some word fun and stimulate your mind by trying this brain teaser from Dr. Small's *The Small Guide to Alzheimer's Disease.*

Spell three words that allow you to go from the word DINER to MENUS by changing only one letter at a time while also forming a proper word at each step.

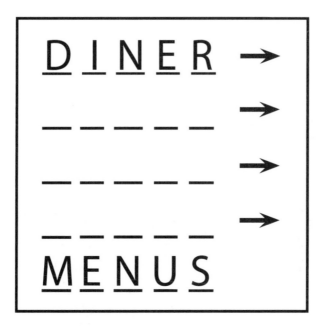

Turn the page for the solution. ➤

BRAIN GAME #17 SOLUTION

(DINER)
MINER
MINES
MINUS
(MENUS)

BRAIN GAME #18

Visual Judgment

Test your visual acuity and mental assumptions by studying the figures below and determining which horizontal line appears longer.

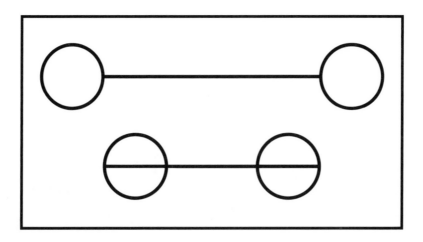

Turn the page for the solution. ➤

BRAIN GAME #18 SOLUTION

**Both horizontal lines are
the same length.**

BRAIN GAME #19

Tricky Division

Here's one that will exercise how well you follow directions.

> # Divide the number 50 by one-half and then add 20.

Turn the page for the solution. ➤

BRAIN GAME #19 SOLUTION

If your answer was 45, then you were not following the directions carefully. The correct answer is 120 as shown in the following formula:

$$50 \div 0.5 = 100$$

$$\text{then } 100 + 20 = 120$$

BRAIN GAME #20

Tell Yourself a Story

If you find yourself too busy to jot down a to-do list for your errands, try visualizing a story that links the tasks together in your mind. For example, if you need to buy eggs and pick up your pants at the cleaners, visualize yourself holding an egg that slips out of your hand and splatters on your pants (reminding you of both errands).

Try out this method for yourself with the following errands:

1. **Take dog to vet**
2. **Get some cash at bank**
3. **Buy stamps at post office**
4. **Pick up flowers for the party**

Turn the page for the solution. ———▶

BRAIN GAME #20 SOLUTION

Dr. Small's example story:

I see myself walking the dog to the vet. On the way, I stop at the ATM, but instead of cash, it spits out stamps with flower displays on them.

What story did you come up with?

BRAIN GAME #21

Word Chain

Here's a fun word game to exercise your brain's left hemisphere.

Begin with the word HAND and then exchange one letter at a time until you get to the word LIME.

Hint: Each change must be a proper word.

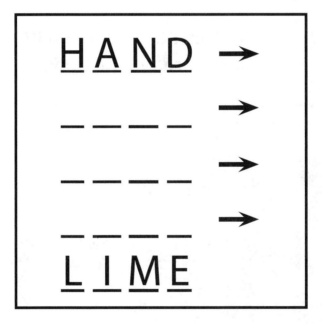

Turn the page for the solution. →

BRAIN GAME #21 SOLUTION

(HAND)

LAND

LANE

LINE

(LIME)

Note: You may have come up with different words in the middle.

BRAIN GAME #22

Matching Socks

You're up early for work and don't want to awaken anyone by turning on the lights; however, you need to get a matching pair of socks from your drawer.

You know there are ten black socks and ten gray socks in the drawer.

How many socks do you need to remove to ensure you have a pair of matching socks?

Turn the page for the solution. ➤

BRAIN GAME #22 SOLUTION

You only need to remove three socks to ensure you have a matching pair.

If your first sock is black and your second sock is gray, the third will make a pair with one of the first two socks.

BRAIN GAME #23

Word Count

Using the letters below, jot down as many words as you can with three or more letters.

Hint: Use each letter only once for each word.

A O M E R A

Turn the page for the solution. ➤

BRAIN GAME #23 SOLUTION

Here are some possible words—you may have found even more words.

AERO, ARE, ARM

ERA

MAR, MARE, MER, MORA, MORE, MORAE

ORE

RAM, REAM, ROAM

BRAIN GAME #24

Mystery Word

Use the following clue to figure out the mystery word.
  Hint: It's often associated with a laboratory.

4N6

Turn the page for the solution. ➔

BRAIN GAME #24 SOLUTION

Forensics

BRAIN GAME #25

Subtraction Equation

Move just one stick to get another correct equation.

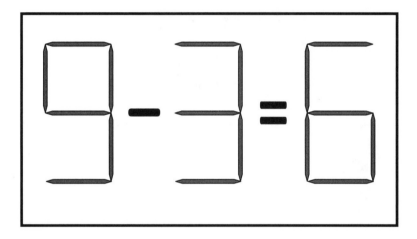

Turn the page for the solution. ➝

BRAIN GAME #25 SOLUTION

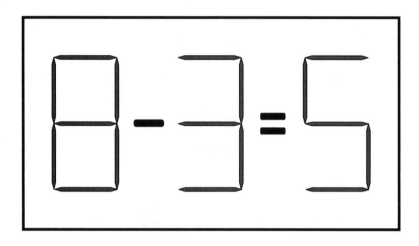

BRAIN GAME #26

Find the Proverb

Figure out the famous proverb from the word jumbles below:

LAL
AHTT
RGTILEST
SI
TON
ODGL

Turn the page for the solution. ➤

BRAIN GAME #26 SOLUTION

ALL THAT GLITTERS IS NOT GOLD.

BRAIN GAME #27

An Unpredictable Riddle

Watch out for your usual mental assumptions to answer the following question:

Matthew McConaughey has a long one. Shelley Long has a short one. Cher and the pope don't use one. What is it?

Turn the page for the solution. ➤

BRAIN GAME #27 SOLUTION

A surname

BRAIN GAME #28

Which Door?

See if you can figure out this fun riddle.

You are trying to escape a room that has three exit doors.

A rattlesnake is waiting for you behind the first door.

A trained assassin is poised behind the second door.

Behind the third door is a lion that has not eaten in years.

Which door is your safest exit strategy?

Turn the page for the solution. ➝

BRAIN GAME #28 SOLUTION

The third door is your best choice.

If the lion had not eaten in years,
it would no longer be alive.

BRAIN GAME #29

Prepare for a Boost

Try this brain teaser to get your cognitive juices flowing.

Write down as many words—made up of three or more letters—as you can think of using the letters below (without repeating a letter in each word):

I A E L S K

Turn the page for the solution. ➤

BRAIN GAME #29 SOLUTION

Dr. Small came up with the following words, but you may have discovered more:

AIL, AILS, AISLE, ALE, ALES, ASK
ELK, ELKS, ELS
ILK, ISLE
KALE, KALES
LAI, LAIS, LAS, LAKE, LAKES, LEA,
LEAS, LEAK, LEAKS, LIKE, LIKES
SAIL, SAKE, SAKI, SALE,
SEA, SEAL, SILK, SKI

BRAIN GAME #30

Famous Saying

All the vowels from a popular proverb have been removed.

Fill in the missing vowels to read the famous saying:

WHN N RM, D S TH RMNS D

Turn the page for the solution. ➤

BRAIN GAME #30 SOLUTION

WHEN IN ROME, DO AS
THE ROMANS DO.

BRAIN GAME #31

Changing Squares

Move just two of the toothpicks below so that instead of five identical squares, you get four identical squares.

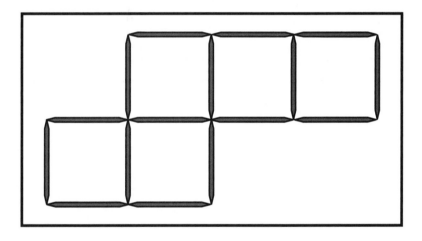

Turn the page for the solution. ━━▶

BRAIN GAME #31 SOLUTION

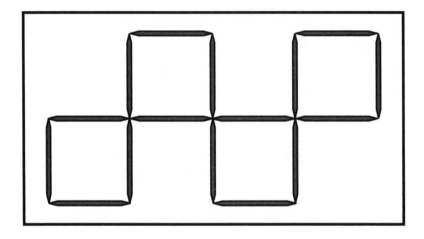

BRAIN GAME #32

Who Is That?

This brain teaser may boggle your mind, but if you use simple deductive reasoning, you will figure it out.

A woman is staring at a photo of someone, and an acquaintance asks her who is in the photo.

The woman says, "I have no sisters, but that woman's mother is my mother's daughter."

Who was the woman in the photo?

Turn the page for the solution. ➤

BRAIN GAME #32 SOLUTION

Her daughter

BRAIN GAME #33

Missing Pieces

Give your brain cells a workout by trying to fill in the missing segments of the letters below to determine the word:

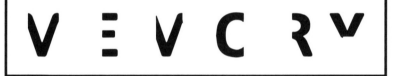

Turn the page for the solution. ➔

BRAIN GAME #33 SOLUTION

The word is "memory."

BRAIN GAME #34

Name That Child

Try to solve this little brain teaser:

Robert's mother had three kids.

The first child's name was April, and the second was called May.

What was the third child's name?

Turn the page for the solution. →

BRAIN GAME #34 SOLUTION

Robert

BRAIN GAME #35

Moving Time

Here's a fun riddle to tweak your frontal lobe circuits.

These days, there are many ways to tell the time of day.

Watches, clocks, and other timepieces come in all shapes and sizes.

Most would agree that a timepiece with the fewest moving parts is a sundial.

Can you think of the timepiece that has the most moving parts?

Turn the page for the solution. ⟶

BRAIN GAME #35 SOLUTION

An hourglass has thousands of
moving parts—that is, grains of sand.

BRAIN GAME #36

What Is It?

Here is another fun riddle that will either make you laugh or groan.

Think of something that satisfies the following three criteria:

1. It has a mouth but cannot eat.
2. It moves but has no legs.
3. It has a bank but no money.

Turn the page for the solution. ➞

BRAIN GAME #36 SOLUTION

A river

BRAIN GAME #37

Shared Feature

Flex your brain cells with this puzzler.

What do these three words have in common?

China

Herb

Polish

Turn the page for the solution. ➤

BRAIN GAME #37 SOLUTION

When the first letter is lowercased, they all have a different meaning.

When not capitalized,

china refers to porcelain tableware;

herb refers to a plant that flavors food;

polish refers to making something shiny.

BRAIN GAME #38

Name the State

Below, you'll find clues to the names of six U.S. states.

The letter indicates the first letter of the state, and the number tells you the number of letters in the state's name.

For example, C10 would be the clue for California.

See how quickly you can come up with the state names.

V7

T5

K6

M11

U4

A7

Turn the page for the solution. ➞

BRAIN GAME #38 SOLUTION

Vermont

Texas

Kansas

Mississippi

Utah

Arizona

How long did it take you to come up with the names? **KEEP PRACTICING.**

BRAIN GAME #39

Grid Work

Here's some grid work that will boost your brain power.

Fill in the grid so that every row and every column, as well as every quadrant, contains the letters W X Y Z.

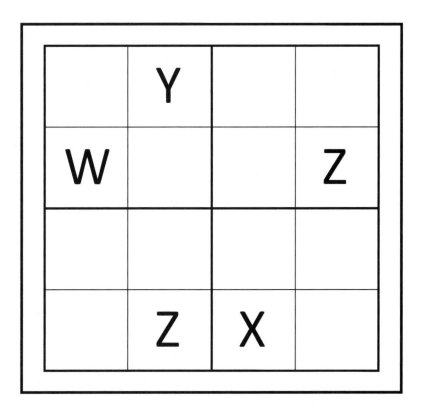

Turn the page for the solution. ➡

BRAIN GAME #39 SOLUTION

Z	Y	W	X
W	X	Y	Z
X	W	Z	Y
Y	Z	X	W

BRAIN GAME #40

Test Your Bearings

You take a one-mile hike due south from your campsite, then turn east and hike another mile.

After that, you turn north and hike another mile and find yourself back at your tent, where there's a bear inside eating your food.

What color is the bear?

Turn the page for the solution. ➤

BRAIN GAME #40 SOLUTION

The bear is white.

The North Pole is the only place where you can hike one mile south, then one mile east, then one mile north, and return to your starting point.

Polar bears are white and the only bears living at the North Pole.

BRAIN GAME #41

Crack the Pattern

Try to figure out the numerical pattern in the grid below and replace the question mark with the correct number.

3	6	5	1
2	1	8	4
3	?	1	9
7	6	1	1

Turn the page for the solution. →

BRAIN GAME #41 SOLUTION

The correct number is 2,
because each of the rows and
columns adds up to 15.

BRAIN GAME #42

What's in Common?

How are the following words similar?

MARCH
CHINA
HAMLET
LENT

Turn the page for the solution. ➤

BRAIN GAME #42 SOLUTION

The words are all *capitonyms*.

Capitonyms are words that change their meaning (and sometimes pronunciation) when the first letter is capitalized.

BRAIN GAME #43

Who's at Home?

A man runs from home for about thirty yards and turns left.

After running the same distance, he turns left again and continues running.

He does this once more and returns home to find two masked men.

> # Who are they?

Turn the page for the solution. ——▶

BRAIN GAME #43 SOLUTION

A catcher and an umpire

BRAIN GAME #44

More Is Less

> **What word becomes shorter when you add two letters to it?**

Turn the page for the solution. ➤

BRAIN GAME #44 SOLUTION

The word is "short."

(Shorter)

BRAIN GAME #45

Not in One Hundred Years

> # What is it that you can find just once in a minute but twice in a moment?

Hint: However, you will never find it in a hundred years?

Turn the page for the solution. ➙

BRAIN GAME #45 SOLUTION

The letter *M*

BRAIN GAME #46

Count on Family

Here's a brain teaser that will warm up your frontal lobe, the area of your brain that controls reasoning and math.

You meet a family made up of two parents and six daughters. Each of the daughters has one brother.

Figure out the total number of people in this family.

Turn the page for the solution. ➡

BRAIN GAME #46 SOLUTION

There are nine (9) people
in this family:

Two (2) parents
Six (6) daughters
One (1) son

BRAIN GAME #47

A to Z by Month

Flex your frontal lobe with the following mental workout.

Without writing them down, say all twelve months of the year in alphabetical order.

If that's too easy for you, try saying them in reverse alphabetical order.

Turn the page for the solution. ➞

BRAIN GAME #47 SOLUTION

Alphabetical order:

April	June
August	March
December	May
February	November
January	October
July	September

Reverse alphabetical order:

September	July
October	January
November	February
May	December
March	August
June	April

BRAIN GAME #48

All or Nothing

Here are two clues to help you figure out a fun but perplexing riddle:

---

1. **Turn it on its side and it is infinite.**
2. **Cut it in half and it's nothing.**

Turn the page for the solution. ➤

BRAIN GAME #48 SOLUTION

The number eight (8).

BRAIN GAME #49

From H to H

> **As quickly as possible, see if you can write down five words that begin and end with the letter *h*.**

If you got five, see if you can think of two more just for fun.

Turn the page for the solution. ➡

BRAIN GAME #49 SOLUTION

Hunch

Hitch

Hutch

Hawkish

Hurrah

Hatch

Huh

BRAIN GAME #50

See the C

Here is a fun mental workout for your visual brain.

As quickly as possible, find the letter C below:

```
O O O O O O O O O O O O O
O O O O O O O O O O O O O
O O O O O O O O O O O O O
O O O O O O O O O O O O O
O O O O O C O O O O O O O
O O O O O O O O O O O O O
O O O O O O O O O O O O O
O O O O O O O O O O O O O
O O O O O O O O O O O O O
```

Turn the page for the solution. ➤

BRAIN GAME #50 SOLUTION

The "C" lost in a sea of "O's" is located in the middle of the fifth row from the top.

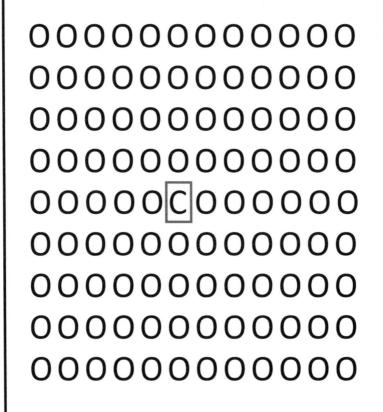

BRAIN GAME #51

Incomplete Thoughts

Here's a fun mental exercise to help you overcome any brain drain.

Below are four incomplete proverbs.

See if you can remember them and complete each sentence.

"Two wrongs don't . . ."
"The pen is mightier than . . ."
"The squeaky wheel gets . . ."
"When the going gets tough . . ."

Turn the page for the solution. ➤

BRAIN GAME #51 SOLUTION

"Two wrongs don't make *a right*."

"The pen is mightier
than *the sword*."

"The squeaky wheel gets *the oil*."

"When the going gets tough,
the tough get going."

BRAIN GAME #52

Heads or Tails?

You flip a coin nine times, and it lands heads up each time.

If you flip that coin one more time, what is the probability that it will land heads up again?

Turn the page for the solution. ➤

BRAIN GAME #52 SOLUTION

50:50

The odds of heads or tails are always 50:50 on a coin toss regardless of the results of previous tosses.

BRAIN GAME #53

Verbal Enigma

Here is a fun riddle that should tweak your frontal lobe's neural circuits.

> # What is something that you can drive but does not have wheels?

Hint: You can also slice it, but it remains whole.

Turn the page for the solution. ➤

BRAIN GAME #53 SOLUTION

A golf ball

BRAIN GAME #54

Memorize a To-Do List

Here's a brain teaser from Dr. Small's book *The Small Guide to Alzheimer's Disease*.

Try thinking up a story that links together items you want to memorize.

For example, you have two errands: buy eggs at the market and pick up your pants at the dry cleaners.

And you are too busy to write them down, so picture yourself carrying an egg that breaks in your hand and stains your slacks—sending them to the cleaners.

Now try to create your own story for remembering the following errands:

---

1. **Pet store—buy dog food**
2. **Bakery—pick up a pie**
3. **Dry cleaner—drop off jacket**

Turn the page for the solution. ➤

BRAIN GAME #54 SOLUTION

Dr. Small's example story:

While walking my dog to the pet store to buy dog food, I got hungry and stopped at a bakery for some pie. My dog leapt for the pie, causing it to go all over my jacket, which then had to go to the dry cleaner.

What story did you come up with?

BRAIN GAME #55

Quick Brain-Building Teaser

Two cab drivers are going the wrong way on a one-way street.

A policeman sees them and doesn't give them a ticket.

> ## Can you think of a plausible explanation?

Turn the page for the solution. ➤

BRAIN GAME #55 SOLUTION

The cab drivers are *walking* the wrong way on a one-way street.

BRAIN GAME #56

Create a story using the words below:

> **Tree**
> **Nun**
> **Newspaper**
> **Basketball**
> **Horse**
> **Rain**
> **Trash Can**

Turn the page for the solution. ———▶

BRAIN GAME #56 SOLUTION

Dr. Small's example story:

A nun riding a horse stops under a tree because it's starting to rain. She covers her head with a newspaper that gets all wet, so she rolls it up and tosses it like a basketball into a trash can.

BRAIN GAME #57

Multiple-Choice Question

People who complete a college education

> **A. Have a higher risk of developing Alzheimer's disease**
>
> **B. Have a lower risk of developing Alzheimer's disease**
>
> **C. Are more arrogant than nongraduates**
>
> **D. None of the above**

Turn the page for the solution. ➤

BRAIN GAME #57 SOLUTION

B. Have a lower risk of developing Alzheimer's disease

Scientists attribute the association between education and lower Alzheimer's risk to the mental stimulation that education provides. But it could also be a result of the fact that educated people are more likely to be aware that habits like exercising and not smoking are good for their health.

BRAIN GAME #58

Photo Recall

Try this exercise for yourself.

Study the photograph below for thirty seconds, noting as much detail as possible, then cover the photo and see if you can answer the questions below.

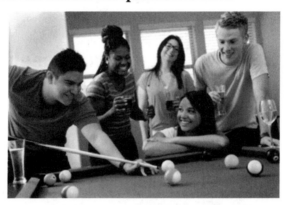

1. How many people are in the photo? How many are women?
2. How many billiard balls are on the table?
3. How many people are holding glasses?
4. Was anyone wearing a striped top?
5. How many windows were there? Drapes or shades?
6. Was everybody standing?
7. How many mugs or glasses? Were there any wineglasses?
8. How many people were touching the pool table?

Turn the page for the solution. ➤

BRAIN GAME #58 SOLUTION

1. Five, three
2. Eight
3. Three
4. Yes—one woman
5. Three—shades
6. No—one woman was kneeling
7. Five mugs or glasses and one is a wineglass
8. Three

BRAIN GAME #59

More Verbal Fluency (i.e., the Ability to Come up with Words)

Set your timer for three minutes, but this time, use the following seven letters to form as many three-or-more-letter words as possible.

A E I O R A M

Turn the page for the solution. ➝

BRAIN GAME #59 SOLUTION

Here are some of the words you
might have come up with:

AERO, ARE, ARM, AIM, ARE, ARM
ERA
IRE
ORE
RAM, RIM RIME, REAM, ROAM
MAR, MARE, MER, MIRA,
MIRE, MORA, MORE, MORAE

Keep practicing and give
yourself more (or less) time.

BRAIN GAME #60

Name That Thing

Rearrange the four letters below to make a word that can be placed into only one of the three categories:

SWPA

A. Plant
B. Tool
C. Insect

Turn the page for the solution. ➡

BRAIN GAME #60 SOLUTION

C. WASP

BRAIN GAME #61

Meaning Mystery

From the following list of words, pick out the two that have the closest meaning.

Over

Climb

Low

Near

Above

Far

A. Low and near

B. Near and far

C. Over and climb

D. Over and above

Turn the page for the solution. ➝

BRAIN GAME #61 SOLUTION

D. Over and above

BRAIN GAME #62

The Next in Line

Complete the sequence by choosing the correct object—A, B, or C.

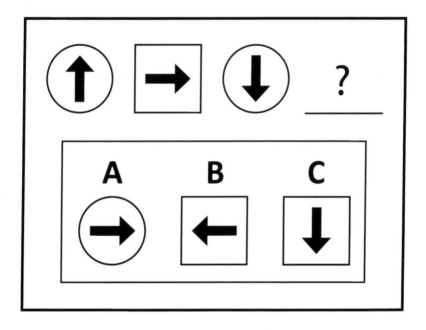

Turn the page for the solution. →

BRAIN GAME #62 SOLUTION

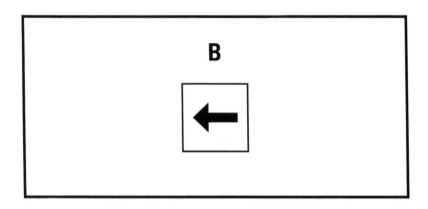

BRAIN GAME #63

Try Sudoku

The goal of Sudoku is to complete a 9 × 9 grid that is sub-divided into nine 3 × 3 boxes.

Some squares will already have numbers in them.

Try to fill in the rest of the squares so that every row, column, and 3 × 3 box contains the numbers 1 to 9 only once.

The difficulty level of the puzzle depends on how many of the digits are already placed in the grid when you start and where they are placed.

The fewer numbers already placed, the harder the puzzle.

	2	7	3	8		5		6
4		5			6	8		1
1		8	4				3	7
3	7	2	1	4		6		
		4		9				2
6		9	5		7	4	8	
8	4		7	6		2		9
2					9			4
	9	6	2	1				8

Turn the page for the solution. ➡

BRAIN GAME #63 SOLUTION

9	2	7	3	8	1	5	4	6
4	3	5	9	7	6	8	2	1
1	6	8	4	5	2	9	3	7
3	7	2	1	4	8	6	9	5
5	8	4	6	9	3	1	7	2
6	1	9	5	2	7	4	8	3
8	4	3	7	6	5	2	1	9
2	5	1	8	3	9	7	6	4
7	9	6	2	1	4	3	5	8

BRAIN GAME #64

Word Jumble

Quickly unscramble the following sets of letters to make eight words.

Then draw lines between the words that go together.

Hint: Your lines should create a number that may remind you of lunchtime.

LEPAP KFRO KRECOR TINSEC
NLSUITE TIRUF IHRCA YLUEBTRFLT

Turn the page for the solution. ——▶

BRAIN GAME #64 SOLUTION

APPLE   FORK   ROCKER   INSECT

UTENSIL FRUIT CHAIR BUTTERFLY

BRAIN GAME #65

Right-Brain Exercise: Counting Squares

Count the number of squares in the figure below.

Hint: Be sure to count the squares within the squares.

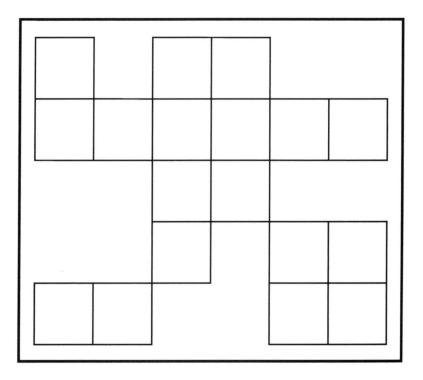

Turn the page for the solution. ➤

BRAIN GAME #65 SOLUTION

21 Squares

BRAIN GAME #66

Left-Brain Exercise: Changing Words

Begin with the word WALL and change one letter at a time until you get to the word FIRM.

  Hint: Each change must be a proper word.

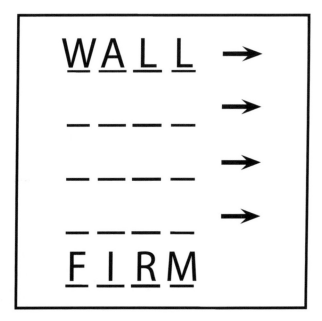

Turn the page for the solution. ➤

BRAIN GAME #66 SOLUTION

(WALL)

WILL

FILL

FILM

(FIRM)

Note: You may have come
up with different words.

BRAIN GAME #67

Numbering Toothpicks

Arrange the three toothpicks below into the number nine (without breaking or bending them).

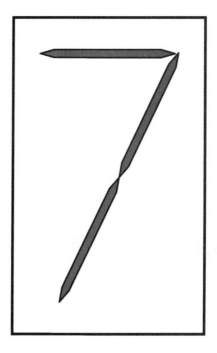

Turn the page for the solution. ➤

BRAIN GAME #67 SOLUTION

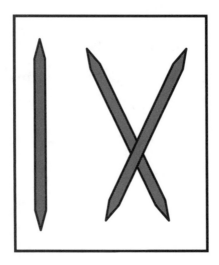

BRAIN GAME #68

Letter Scramble

Try to come up with as many words as you can from the following letters.

Hint: Use each letter only once in each word.

I R N A B

Turn the page for the solution. →

BRAIN GAME #68 SOLUTION

I, IN

RA, RAN, RIB, RAIN

NA, NAN, NAB

A, AN, AIR

BA, BAN, BAR, BIN,
BARN, BRAN, BRAIN

BRAIN GAME #69

Jigsaw Brain Break

Keep your right brain in shape today.
Which piece fits in the puzzle:

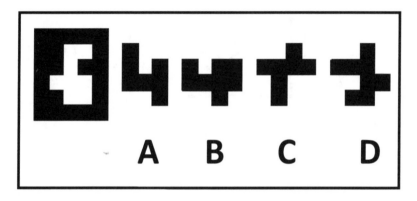

A   B   C   D

Turn the page for the solution. ➔

BRAIN GAME #69 SOLUTION

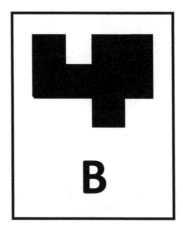

B

BRAIN GAME #70

Sorting Words

The brain naturally organizes information into categories to make memory more efficient.

It's easier to remember two fruits and two vegetables than four individual items.

Strengthen your sorting skills by identifying the three categories of the nine items below:

Chicken
Pliers
Magazine
Wrench
Novel
Yogurt
Biography
Salmon
Vice

Turn the page for the solution. ⟶

BRAIN GAME #70 SOLUTION

Tools:

Pliers   Vice

Wrench

Reading Materials:

Magazine   Biography

Novel

Edibles:

Chicken   Salmon

Yogurt

BRAIN GAME #71

Visual Connecting

Here is another brain workout to enhance your right brain's visual-spatial skills and your frontal lobe's ability to split your attention between two mental tasks.

In the figure below, draw a continuous line that connects the number 1 to the letter A, then A to 2, then 2 to B, then B to 3, and so on until you can no longer continue the numerical or the alphabetical sequence.

Hint: If you get this right, give yourself a star.

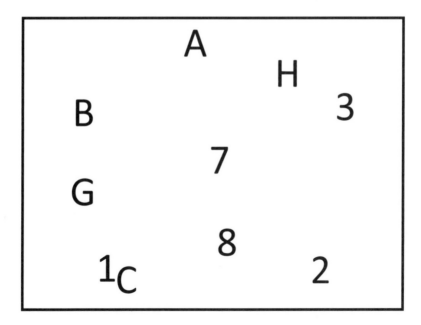

Turn the page for the solution. ➤

BRAIN GAME #71 SOLUTION

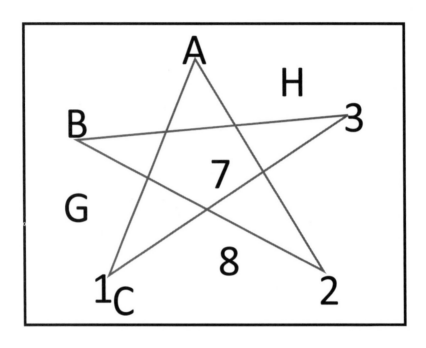

BRAIN GAME #72

Finding Colors

Rearrange the letters to find the four colors mixed up below.

Hint: Only one is a primary color.

RAIGET

ENOLYL

OVGOEN

LEWRE

Turn the page for the solution. ➞

BRAIN GAME #72 SOLUTION

GREEN
ORANGE
VIOLET
YELLOW (primary color)

BRAIN GAME #73

Letter Scramble

Using the letters below, write down as many words as you can with three or more letters.

Hint: Each letter can only be used once in each word.

I M R O A E

Turn the page for the solution. ➞

BRAIN GAME #73 SOLUTION

IRE

MAR, MARE, MIRE, MORE

RAM, REAM, RIM, RIME, ROAM

OAR, ORE

ARM, ARMOR

EAR

Note: You may find more. Try again with more time or less time.

BRAIN GAME #74

Jigsaw Brain Break

Your right brain needs a little more of a workout.
Which piece fits in the puzzle?

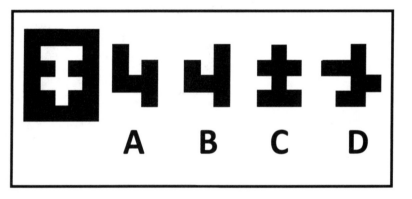

Turn the page for the solution. ➔

BRAIN GAME #74 SOLUTION

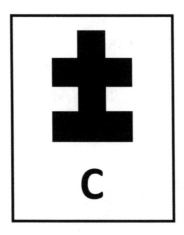

BRAIN GAME #75

Proverb

All the vowels have been removed from the following proverb, and the remaining letters have been clustered into groups of three or four letters each.

Replace the vowels and reveal the proverb.

> **TWH**
> **DSRB**
> **TTRT**
> **HNN**

Turn the page for the solution. ⟶

BRAIN GAME #75 SOLUTION

TWO HEADS ARE BETTER THAN ONE.

BRAIN GAME #76

Letter Scramble

Try to come up with as many words as you can (two or more letters) from the following letters:

OGEUNRY

Turn the page for the solution. ——▶

BRAIN GAME #76 SOLUTION

ON, OR, OY, ONE, ORE, ORG

GEN, GUN, GUY, GYN, GONE,
GORE, GREY, GONER

EON

UN

NU, NUG

RUE, RUN, RUG, RUNG, ROUGE

YO, YON, YOU, YOUNG, YOUNGER

BRAIN GAME #77

Hypothetical Country

A large nation has an overpopulation problem.

For socioeconomic reasons, families prefer to have boys over girls, and most families continue to have children until the birth of a son.

> **If we assume the same probability for girls and boys to be born, what will be the ratio of girls to boys in this country after ten generations?**

Turn the page for the solution. ⟶

BRAIN GAME #77 SOLUTION

The ratio of girls to boys
will still be 50:50.

The odds of having a boy or girl will
remain the same even if all families
adopted the strategy of no more
births after their first son is born.

BRAIN GAME #78

Visual Connecting #2

In the figure below, draw a continuous line connecting the first odd number 1 to the first letter of the alphabet A, then to 3 (the next odd number) and to the next letter of the alphabet B, then 5 to C, and so on until you can no longer continue the sequences.

Hint: If you succeed, you will have drawn a recognizable structure.

Turn the page for the solution. ⟶

BRAIN GAME #78 SOLUTION

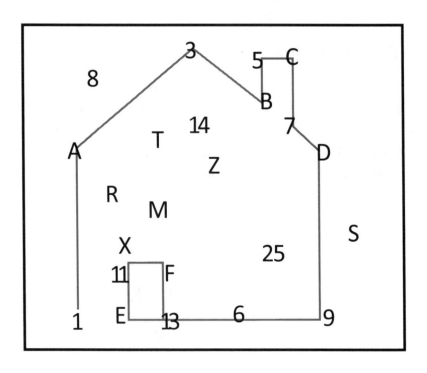

BRAIN GAME #79

Sequence Recognition

See if you can recognize the incomplete sequence below and add four lines to complete it.

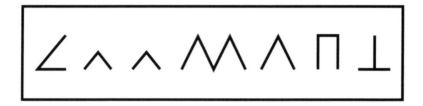

Turn the page for the solution. ➡

BRAIN GAME #79 SOLUTION

Correctly placing four lines gives you the sequence of alphabet letters from Z to T upside down:

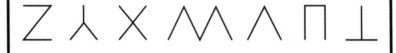

BRAIN GAME #80

Odd One Out

Keep your sorting skills in top form.

Pick out the word below that does not belong in the category suggested by all the other words.

Hint: You will need to unscramble each word first to identify the main category.

ANTK

PJEE

XITA

UNBMARIES

BREOBM

Turn the page for the solution. ➜

BRAIN GAME #80 SOLUTION

The correct answer is

XITA (TAXI).

All the other unscrambled words are military vehicles (TANK, JEEP, SUBMARINE, BOMBER).

BRAIN GAME #81

Finicky Frank

Frank has very eccentric tastes.

He is a big fan of football but hates rugby.

He very much likes beer but despises ale.

He drives a Ferrari but wouldn't be caught dead in a Lamborghini.

> ## Based on Frank's finicky tastes, would he prefer skiing or cycling?

Turn the page for the solution. ➤

BRAIN GAME #81 SOLUTION

Frank would prefer skiing, since he only likes words that contain double letters.

BRAIN GAME #82

Sequence Recognition

Here is another sequence that includes verbal skills, visual skills, and reasoning abilities involving pattern recognition.

Figure out which tile completes the sequence.

Ilk	Here	Gap
Fine	Elf	Dine
Con	Bail	

Apt	Alps	Coil
A	**B**	**C**

Din	Nail	Irk
D	**E**	**F**

Turn the page for the solution. ➞

BRAIN GAME #82 SOLUTION

Tile "A," which contains the word "apt," completes the sequence.

APT

The first letter of the word in each tile is in reverse alphabetical order ("I" from "Ilk" is after "H" in "Here," etc.).

The words also alternate from three to four letters.

BRAIN GAME #83

Meal-Planning Brain Game

You mention to your boss that he and his wife should come by your new place for dinner sometime, and he says they are available that very night.

You do not have time to go to the market, so you have to use what's already in your refrigerator and pantry.

Because your boss is a fitness enthusiast, you want to impress him by making a health-conscious meal.

You know you have enough vegetables to prepare a salad and frozen yogurt for dessert, but you have to improvise the entrée.

Once home, you find you have the following ingredients below.

As quickly as possible, check off the ingredients you'll use to create a main course, and then write the name of that course at the bottom.

___ Ground beef	___Onions	___Whole milk
___ Chicken breasts	___Butter	___Sugar
___ Mushrooms	___Olive oil	___Bacon
___ Tomatoes	___Cornflakes	___Mayonnaise
___ Cheddar cheese	___Whole-wheat pasta	___Hamburger buns
___ Whipping cream	___Cream of mushroom soup	
___ Frozen cheese ravioli		

Main course _____

Turn the page for the solution. ➔

BRAIN GAME #83 SOLUTION

A tasty and nutritious entrée would have been grilled chicken breasts served with whole wheat spaghetti and fresh tomato sauce with onions and mushrooms in it.

Note: If you used the ground beef, buns, cheddar cheese, and bacon to make bacon cheeseburgers, they probably tasted good, but you didn't impress your boss with your healthy eating.

BRAIN GAME #84

Exercise Brain Teaser

Unscramble the letters below to find the exercise that focuses more on strength training than aerobic conditioning.

GOJNGGI

USPPHUS

MGMSINWI

AKLGINW

CCLINGY

Turn the page for the solution. ➡

BRAIN GAME #84 SOLUTION

If you correctly unscrambled the four words, you'd see that the second word, PUSHUPS, is the correct answer, since JOGGING, SWIMMING, WALKING, and CYCLING are all forms of aerobic conditioning.

BRAIN GAME #85

Right-Brain Toothpick Teaser Exercise(s)

Here's a spatial exercise to keep your visual neural circuits flexible.

Take five toothpicks and arrange them so they are all touching and display the number 5.

Bonus: Then rearrange the five toothpicks so they display an unlucky number.

Turn the page for the solution. ➜

BRAIN GAME #85 SOLUTION

Here is how your toothpicks should have been arranged so they are all touching and display the number 5:

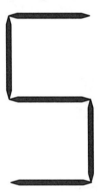

Here is how your toothpicks should have been arranged so they display an unlucky number:

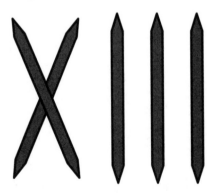

BRAIN GAME #86

Word-Generation Exercise

> Get a pen and paper, and
> then make a list of as many
> animals that begin with the
> letter *P* as you can think of.

Turn the page for the solution. ⟶

BRAIN GAME #86 SOLUTION

Dr. Small's *P* animals:

Parakeet
Parrot
Partridge
Peacock
Pelican
Penguin
Pheasant
Pigeon
Platypus
Porcupine
Possum
Puma
Python

What did you come up with? Can you think of more animals with more time? Or in less time? Try again.

BRAIN GAME #87

Remembering Nonvisual Names

When trying to remember a complicated name, or one that doesn't immediately bring an image to mind, try altering the name or its spelling slightly. For example,

- To visualize the name Tyler, see her working as a tailor.
- For Paul, visualize him on top of a pole.

Now alter these names so you can generate a visual image.

Tom Siegel

Olivia Newton

Rosa Flores

Turn the page for the solution. ⟶

BRAIN GAME #87 SOLUTION

Here are some of Dr. Small's suggestions:

- **For *Tom Siegel*, visualize him playing a tom-tom drum with a sea gull on his shoulder.**
- **For *Olivia Newton*, see her eating a Fig Newton with an olive on top (or you could just imagine her singing with Olivia Newton John).**
- **See *Rosa Flores* dropping a large vase of roses on the floor.**

What did you come up with?

BRAIN GAME #88

Everyday Task-Sorting Exercise

When our brains organize information into categories, it makes it simpler to recall. When going to the market, it's easier to remember to buy two kinds of cereals and two fruits rather than four items that are not sorted into categories.

Strengthen your sorting skills by identifying the four categories for the following sixteen items and then sort them into their proper categories:

Orange	Grapes
Rugby	Beagle
Sonata	Track
Avocado	Wrestling
Tennis	Opera
Jazz	Poodle
Apple	Terrier
Dachshund	Concerto

Turn the page for the solution. ➤

BRAIN GAME #88 SOLUTION

Sports:

Rugby   Track

Tennis   Wrestling

Dogs:

Dachshund   Poodle

Beagle   Terrier

Fruits:

Orange   Apple

Avocado   Grapes

Music:

Sonata   Opera

Jazz   Concerto

BRAIN GAME #89

Create a narrative to remember the following seven words, some related, some unrelated.

Window
Bed
Cloud
Pillow
Lightning
Spider
Cup

Turn the page for the solution. ➤

BRAIN GAME #89 SOLUTION

Here is Dr. Small's suggestion for a story:

I get into bed and see a spider on my pillow. I scoop it up with my teacup and set it outside on the windowsill just as a dark cloud bursts with lightning and thunder.

What did you come up with?

BRAIN GAME #90

Another Word-Generation Exercise

> **Get a pen and paper, and then jot down seven animals that begin with the letter _D_.**

Turn the page for the solution. ➛

BRAIN GAME #90 SOLUTION

Dr. Small's *D* animals:

Deer
Dingo
Dog
Dolphin
Donkey
Dove
Duck

**What did you come up with?
Can you think of more animals with
more time? Or in less time? Try again.**

FREE BRAIN GAMES WEBSITES

- **BrainBashers:** www.brainbashers.com
- **Brain Den:** www.brainden.com
- **Braingle:** www.braingle.com
- **The Grey Labyrinth:** www.greylabyrinth.com
- **PedagoNet:** www.pedagonet.com/brain/brainers.html
- **Sharp Brains:** www.sharpbrains.com
- **Syvum:** www.syvum.com/teasers
- **Tricky Riddles:** www.trickyriddles.com
- **The Ultimate Puzzle Site:** www.puzzle.dse.nl

PART 2:

HEALTH CARE FOR A BETTER BRAIN

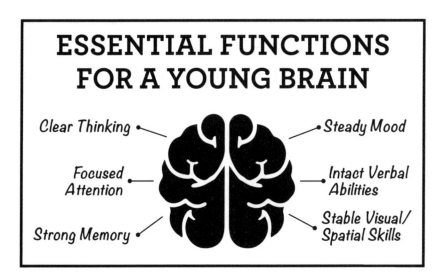

ESSENTIAL FUNCTIONS FOR A YOUNG BRAIN

Clear Thinking

Focused Attention

Strong Memory

Steady Mood

Intact Verbal Abilities

Stable Visual/ Spatial Skills

THE BASICS

- Your doctor can address your health concerns and answer your questions about medical issues and lifestyle habits that affect your health.

- Bringing all your medicines (or a list of them) to your doctor appointment can help make sure that your prescription and over-the-counter drugs are not causing any memory side effects, and always discuss anything new you want to start taking.

- If you have high blood pressure or cholesterol, diabetes, or another chronic medical illness, your doctor's suggestions may be crucial for optimal brain health.

- Patients with Alzheimer's dementia can temporarily benefit from antidementia medicines that help maintain a higher level of functioning longer.

- Hormones and supplements have been used to treat age-related memory loss, but long-term benefits have not been confirmed.

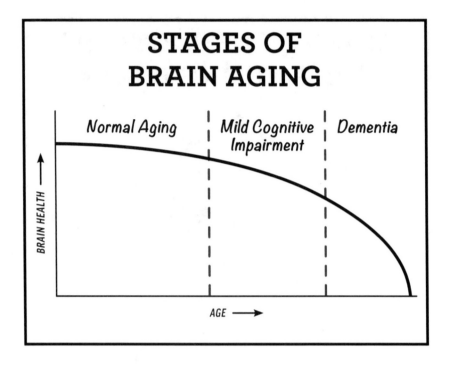

COMMON SYMPTOMS OF NORMAL BRAIN AGING

- Forgetting names and faces
- Not remembering where you put things
- Failing to recall an appointment or plan
- Forgetting a word or name you should know that is on the tip of your tongue

SYMPTOMS OF DEMENTIA

- Memory loss
- Difficulties in reasoning
- Disorientation, getting lost
- Language difficulties such as word-finding

- Misplacing things
- Mood or personality changes
- Showing less interest or initiative
- Trouble completing familiar tasks like cooking or cleaning

POSSIBLE CAUSES OF DEMENTIA

Although most dementias are chronic and progressive, sometimes a treatable medical cause is uncovered, which reverses some, or occasionally all, the symptoms. There are hundreds of different causes of dementia. Below are some of the more common ones and examples.

Possible Cause	Examples
Medical illness	Pneumonia, heart failure, cardiac arrhythmia, thyroid abnormalities, anemia, cancer, liver disease, lung disease, kidney failure, infections, metabolic disturbances, vitamin B12 or folate deficiency, autoimmune disease
Medications	Sedatives, antidepressants, over-the-counter sleep medicines, antihistamines, steroids, pain medicines

Possible Cause	Examples
Neurodegenerative disorders	Lewy bodies (abnormal brain protein deposits), frontotemporal dementia, Parkinson's disease, normal pressure hydrocephalus (excess brain fluid), vascular disease, Down syndrome
Psychiatric disorders	Depression, anxiety
Other conditions	Head injury, toxic exposures

DOCTORS WHO CARE FOR MEMORY-IMPAIRED PATIENTS

Because of the shortage of neurologists and geriatric psychiatrists, many primary care doctors have developed expertise in diagnosing and treating dementia. Then again, certain clinical situations are best addressed by particular specialists.

Primary care physicians. For typical cases that do not present in unusual ways, internists and family practitioners who have an interest in cognitive problems are able to effectively diagnose and treat patients with dementia.

Geriatric psychiatrists. These specialists are well equipped to care for patients who have symptoms of depression, anxiety, personality change, or psychosis that often develop along with their cognitive symptoms. Geriatric psychiatrists can also be helpful if psychological conflicts emerge among family members.

Neurologists. Any patient experiencing a cognitive decline along with a neurological condition such as Parkinson's disease or Huntington's disease might wish to seek a consultation from a neurologist.

Geriatricians. Patients with multiple medical problems or gait instability, as well as those aged eighty years or older, may benefit from seeing a geriatric internist.

HEALTH CARE CHECKLIST

- Prepare your questions in advance and bring them to your doctor appointment.
- Copy articles about relevant health topics that may be confusing and review them with your doctor.
- Bring in your medicines (or a list of them) so your doctor can review them and help you avoid harmful drug interactions. This should include prescription medicines, over-the-counter pills, and supplements.
- Discuss nonmedical issues that relate to your health, including exercise, diet, and stress.
- If blood tests or diagnostic studies are performed, be proactive and call for your results if you don't hear from your doctor's office first.

- If you are not comfortable with your doctor's recommendations, seek another opinion.

ORGANIZATIONS FOR FINDING A DOCTOR FOR COGNITIVE ISSUES

The websites of the following organizations include links that can guide you to doctors in your area:

Alzheimer's Association (www.alz.org). This national organization provides information on services, programs, publications, and local chapters.

Alzheimer's Foundation of America (www.alzfdn.org). A nonprofit foundation supporting strategies that help lighten the burden and improve the quality of life of Alzheimer's patients and their caregivers.

American Academy of Neurology (www.aan .com). This professional organization advances the art and science of neurology, thereby promoting the best possible care for patients with neurological disorders.

American Association for Geriatric Psychiatry (www.aagponline.org). A professional organization that is dedicated to enhancing the mental health and well-being of older adults through education and research.

American Geriatrics Society (www
.americangeriatrics.org). A professional
association that provides assistance in
identifying local geriatric physician referrals.

American Psychiatric Association (www
.psychiatry.org). A medical specialty society
that works to ensure that mental disorders
are accurately diagnosed and receive effective
treatments.

PART 3:

WHAT *YOU* CAN DO TO PROTECT YOUR BRAIN

COMMON PSYCHOLOGICAL REACTIONS TO AGE-RELATED MEMORY LOSS

Fear: "I'm losing my mind—I'm going to end up in a nursing home."

Denial: "All my friends are forgetful at my age—there's nothing wrong with me."

Anger: "I get so mad when I can't find the right word."

Self-pity: "Why me? I'm too young to have these problems."

Guilt: "I should have taken better care of myself."

Depression: "I'm nothing without my memory—why should I bother going on like this?"

LOWER STRESS TO PROTECT YOUR BRAIN

- Try meditation to reduce stress and lift your mood.
- Get regular physical exercise to boost brain circulation and endorphin levels.

- Limit multitasking to improve efficiency, diminish distractions, and bolster memory performance.
- Experiment with proven stress-busting activities like yoga and tai chi.
- Try laughing to gain perspective on everyday worries.
- Learn strategies for getting a good night's sleep.
- Get organized and reduce clutter for a greater sense of control.
- Try acupuncture to help reduce pain and stress.
- Keep a positive attitude and strong social relationships.
- Learn to ask for help.

HONE YOUR STRESS DETECTOR

The next time you are people watching, focus on someone and take note of any body language, gestures, or facial expressions that convey whether that person is under stress. Do you notice a wrinkled brow? Is the woman at the next table tapping her foot or restlessly looking around? Does that businessman walking by seem to be late for an appointment? Is he constantly checking his watch? The more you practice, the easier it will become to distinguish between those who seem calm and those who seem stressed out.

Once you're confident in identifying these cues, turn your attention to yourself. Are you sending off stressed-out signals? Are your muscles tense? Are you twirling your hair or pacing without realizing it? If so, take some deep breaths and consider what might be gnawing at you.

TALKING TO YOURSELF REDUCES STRESS

Almost all of us talk to ourselves from time to time. Sometimes we do it when we're happy; other times when we're tense. Talking out loud to ourselves has been shown to lower stress levels and calm us down.

Recent studies indicate that if you address yourself by name in the third person, your self-talk is even more effective in reducing anxiety and building confidence.

Here are a few examples of helpful self-chats for various situations:

- **Speaking in public:** "Remember to make eye contact, Gary, and speak clearly."
- **Applying for a job:** "They'd be lucky to hire someone like Shirley. Shirley has the talent and the ability."
- **Competing in sports:** "Focus on your forehand, Susan. It's your best tennis stroke."
- **Proposing marriage:** "You know she loves you, Steve. She will definitely say yes."

A QUICK AND EASY STRESS-BUSTER

Meditation, yoga, and other stress-reduction exercises help shift our minds away from stress-related, brain-damaging neural activity to more mindful, relaxed, and brain-protective states. Take a couple minutes to try this exercise for a quick mindfulness boost:

- Sit in a comfortable chair, place your feet flat on the floor, and allow them to point slightly outward.
- Rest your hands on your thighs with your palms facing up and close your eyes.
- Take some deep, slow breaths in through your nose, exhaling through your mouth.
- Feel your body relax as your mind grows peaceful.
- Continue inhaling and exhaling for another minute or two, then open your eyes.

STRESS-REDUCTION BREAK

Lie down or sit in a comfortable chair. Take a few deep, slow breaths and then close your eyes. Begin to relax each muscle group in your body, starting with your toes and feet. Release any tension you are holding there, and as you continue breathing slowly, let that sense of relaxation move up through your calves and into your thighs. Next, let the relaxation spread through your pelvis and abdomen. Gradually relax the muscles in your chest, arms, and hands. As you next relax your shoulders and neck, you may wish to move them around a bit to release any tension there. Now relax your jaw and facial muscles.

Finally, take another deep breath, exhale, and open your eyes. Your body will feel relaxed, and your mind will be tranquil. This is a very effective way to quickly de-stress any time of day.

PRACTICE YOUR MENTAL FOCUS SKILLS

Many people find that when they improve their ability to pay attention, their recall skills improve almost immediately. Try these easy exercises and see how well you do.

As you watch a movie or TV show, make a conscious effort to pay attention to particular details. You can choose to focus your attention on props, hairdos, wardrobe, or whatever you like. Test yourself the next day to see how much detail you recall. If you saw the show with a friend or your spouse, dazzle them with your attention skills by casually mentioning the grand piano in the room where the butler dropped the tray.

The next time you have a conversation with someone, try to pay particular attention to what that person is saying. Make a mental note of some small detail, particularly one that you think the person might not expect you to remember—it could be where she plans to have dinner that night or what time she has to go to the dentist. See if you remember the detail the next day. If so, give that person a call or send her a text to ask how it went. Mastering this exercise not only boosts your memory ability but also improves your social skills and can make you more popular.

HEALTHY RELATIONSHIPS FOR BETTER BRAIN HEALTH

- Remain involved with friends and family, because social bonds strengthen brain cell connections.

- Engage in daily discussions about topics of interest to keep your neural circuits agile. Conversations are mental calisthenics that bolster neural networks.

- Spend time with health-conscious people. Doing so promotes your own brain and body health, because good habits are contagious.

- Try to let go of toxic relationships so you have more time to spend with people you truly like.

- Practice paying full attention when you listen to others. Try not to interrupt or misinterpret their feelings.

- Try to share your feelings without criticizing, and let your friends know you understand how they feel. Empathy is a powerful social skill that can be learned and developed.

- Use humor to help diffuse tension and become closer to others, but make sure the timing and situation are right. Avoid negative jokes that express anger or resentment.

FINE-TUNE YOUR LISTENING SKILLS

One reason that people often do not connect to one another is that they don't focus their attention during conversations. Here is an exercise that can strengthen your ability to avoid distractions and heighten your listening skills. It's best to attempt this exercise with a close friend or partner. It doesn't take much time but can really enhance your attention and let the other person know you care about what they're saying.

Ask your partner to discuss an issue that has personal meaning—perhaps a recent problem, a long-term challenge, or an upcoming event. Tell your partner to focus on feelings and avoid criticism, and you should do the same when it's your turn to talk. Avoiding personal attacks will reduce defensiveness and help the listener focus more on understanding. Set your timer for two minutes while your partner talks.

As you listen, maintain eye contact and try not to interrupt—this will help you pay attention. Your mind may wander, or you may have an emotional reaction to the conversation, but try to ignore those distractions and bring your focus back to listening. After your two minutes of listening, reset your timer for two minutes and switch roles so that you are the speaker and your partner is the listener. You may wish to continue discussing the same topic or pick an entirely different one. While speaking, continue to avoid criticism and focus on expressing your feelings.

The last step is to discuss how each of you felt about the exercise. Did it make you feel closer? Was it frustrating? Was it exhilarating?

HOW EMPATHIC ARE YOU?

Some people are born more empathic than others. They're better at understanding someone else's feelings and perspectives and are more effective at conveying their understanding. Answer the following questions to get an idea of your current empathic abilities.

- **Do you sometimes get bored when people talk about their feelings?** Yes or no?

- **Is it difficult to place another person's interests ahead of your own?** Yes or no?

- **Do you prefer distancing yourself from friends who upset you rather than discussing your differences?** Yes or no?

- **Are you uncomfortable talking about your feelings?** Yes or no?

- **Do you tend to change topics in a conversation when it gets too personal?** Yes or no?

- **When you are upset, do you prefer to be alone rather than discuss it with a friend?** Yes or no?

If you answered yes to one or more of the questions, then focusing on developing better empathy skills might improve your social connections and brain health.

Even if you scored well on this brief quiz, building empathy skills can still enhance your relationships and be worth the effort.

BRIEF EMPATHY EXERCISE

Your friend tells you about the following upsetting situation:

"My husband is really getting to me. I can barely look him in the eye I'm so angry. I can't stand that he spends more time with his golf buddies than with me, and he forgot to get me a present on my birthday. I really do love him, but we don't have any romance in our lives."

Before proceeding, spend a moment considering how you might respond.

Here are several possibilities:

Offer unsolicited advice. "You're crazy to criticize him. I know he loves you, and no relationship is perfect." This kind of unsolicited advice is usually unwelcome. If you lecture your friend, she probably won't feel supported. The desire to fix somebody else's problem often stems from our own anxiety that the conflict is causing us.

Share your own experience. "I know exactly what you're feeling. My ex-husband was really a jerk—his job was always more important than our marriage." You may be trying to help by relating your similar experience, but the timing could be wrong. Instead of showing empathy, you are switching the focus to your own problems and suggesting that your marital solution could be right for your friend.

Reflect and mirror. "I didn't know you felt that way. I can see that you are upset and angry. Tell me more about what's going on." This response is much more empathic. Repeating back how your friend feels indicates that you are listening, and it shows your interest and concern.

A GOOD NIGHT'S SLEEP OPTIMIZES BRAIN HEALTH

Avoid daytime naps. These may be invigorating but can lead to less tiredness at bedtime. To break the afternoon-nap habit, try walking or exercising during that time to better sleep at night.

Limit evening liquids and caffeine. Drinking liquids in the evening may cause you to awaken in the night if your bladder calls. If you are sensitive to caffeine, avoid coffee, tea, Cola sodas, or even chocolate, which can keep you awake due to their caffeine content.

Create a restful environment. Make sure your bedding, pillows, and sheets are as comfortable as possible. Keep the bedroom quiet, dark, and cool.

Take it easy in the evening. Some people have trouble settling down after watching an exciting movie or sports event, so try to avoid too much mental stimulation before bedtime.

Use relaxation methods. Deep breathing, imagery, meditation, or anything that relaxes you can help you drift off to sleep. Once you're in bed, keep your body in a comfortable and still position.

Train your brain to sleep. The following technique has worked for several of my patients: get into bed at the same time every night, and don't eat or watch television while in bed. Take a few moments to get comfortable and relax. If you have not fallen asleep after twenty minutes, get up, leave the bedroom, and either read a book, listen to music, or watch television. Once you begin feeling tired, go back to bed and try to sleep again. If you're still not asleep in twenty minutes, get up and leave the bedroom again. Return to bed when sleepy and attempt to fall asleep for another twenty minutes. You may need to continue this method throughout the night, but make sure you don't nap the next day. After sticking to this strategy for a day or two, many people are able to train their brains to sleep through the night.

STAYING PHYSICALLY FIT FOR A YOUNGER BRAIN

- Try to maintain your physical fitness program at every age—brain benefits have been documented in twentysomethings as well as eighty-year-olds.

- Keep a regular aerobic routine. It will enlarge your hippocampal memory center in just six months.

- Determine your baseline to help you understand where to begin your fitness program.

- Make exercise fun so it becomes a habit. Try keeping it social, competitive, and creative—soon your brain and body will crave it.

- Adjust your program to accommodate for any injuries so they don't hold you back.

- Protect yourself from traumatic brain injury— wear a helmet and avoid bumping your head.

- Incorporate strength and balance training. While regular aerobic exercise is essential, strength and balance training offers additional brain-health benefits.

- Integrate exercise into your daily lifestyle by taking the stairs, walking briskly between appointments, and engaging in regular stretching and exercise breaks throughout the day.

TIPS TO MAKE EXERCISE FUN

- **Make it social.** Enjoying conversation while working out with friends benefits both your body and your brain.

- **Compete.** The heated excitement of tennis, volleyball, and other competitive sports engages our brains and keeps us coming back. If you'd prefer not to compete against others, compete against yourself by continually challenging yourself to improve your times or increase your number of repetitions.

- **Add brain games.** Do puzzles and brain teasers while on the stationary bike or treadmill: new research shows that you get more out of mental workouts when your heart is pumping hard at the same time.

- **Shake it up.** Your brain loves variety, so don't just stick with one routine or sport.

- **Get outdoors.** Swap the treadmill for the outdoors so you can enjoy the scenery and explore new surroundings while you exercise.

EATING WELL FOR A YOUNGER BRAIN

- Make your diet delicious and nutritious. In just two weeks, you can alter your brain's neural circuits and make it easier to stick with your diet and enjoy it.

- Some people can become addicted to certain foods or too much food, so it's important to recognize and avoid anything that might trigger you to overeat.

- Eat at least five servings of a variety of colorful fruits and vegetables every day to fight off your brain's oxidative stress.

- Omega-3 fats from fish, nuts, and flaxseed are natural anti-inflammatories and protect brain cells from age-related damage.

- Being overweight or obese is bad for your brain, so if weight is a concern, limit your caloric intake and increase your activity level.

- Combining healthy proteins and carbohydrates at every meal and snack will boost your energy and keep you satisfied longer.

- Protect your brain by cutting back on refined sugars in your diet. This will lower your risk of becoming overweight or obese and for developing diabetes.

- Caffeine and alcohol are good for your brain if consumed in moderation.

YOUR BRAIN-HEALTH DIET

Changing how you eat to keep your brain young involves following a few guidelines:

- **Eat small meals throughout the day.** Have breakfast, a midmorning snack, lunch, a midafternoon snack, and dinner to avoid getting too hungry at any one time.

- **Combine healthy proteins and carbohydrates at every meal.** This combination provides immediate energy from the carbs and sustained satiety from the proteins.

- **Get adequate hydration, vitamins, and minerals.** Drink several 8-ounce glasses of water, along with 1 multivitamin and 1,000 milligrams of omega-3 fatty acid (fish oil) each day.
- **Eat healthy omega-3 fats.** Eat fish at least twice each week and/or nuts and flaxseed to help control inflammation.
- **Include antioxidant fruits and vegetables.** Colorful fruits and green leafy vegetables fight oxidation and provide fiber to promote digestion.
- **Minimize omega-6 fats, refined sugars, and processed foods.** A steak or cookie once in a while is OK, but don't make a habit of it.
- **Practice portion control.** Try splitting entrées at restaurants and putting less on your plate at home.

TEN NUTRITION TIPS TO KEEP YOUR MIND SHARP

1. **Set realistic goals.** If you make your diet too restrictive, it will be hard to stick to. Avoid fad diets and set reasonable goals so you can maintain your diet.
2. **Control portions.** Obesity puts you at risk for diabetes, Alzheimer's, and other illnesses that threaten brain health, so limit your caloric intake.
3. **Eat frequent small meals.** Rather than fasting all day and splurging at dinner, eat smaller

portions at breakfast, lunch, dinner, and two between-meal snacks.

4. **Combine proteins and carbs.** At each meal or snack, combine healthy proteins and carbohydrates for an energy boost (carbs) and sustained satiety (proteins).

5. **Eat fruits and vegetables.** Eating five servings of fruits and vegetables each day will protect your brain cells from the wear and tear of oxidative stress.

6. **Consume omega-3 fatty acids.** These healthy fats protect your brain from inflammation. Fish, nuts, or flaxseed are excellent sources.

7. **Limit refined sugar and processed foods.** Minimizing these foods will lower your risk for obesity, diabetes, and other illnesses that can damage your brain.

8. **Moderate caffeine use.** Moderate use of coffee and tea is associated with a lower risk for Alzheimer's disease and other forms of dementia.

9. **Spice it up.** Flavor your food with herbs and spices for additional antioxidant power to protect your brain and allow you to use less salt. Lowering salt intake will help you avoid brain-damaging high blood pressure.

10. **Know your triggers.** Certain foods trigger some people to overeat. Whether it's chocolate, ice cream, or bread, know your triggers and avoid them.

EXAMPLES OF ANTIOXIDANT FRUITS AND VEGETABLES

Fruits:	Vegetables:
Avocados	Alfalfa sprouts
Blackberries	Artichokes
Blueberries	Beets
Cantaloupe	Bell peppers
Cherries	Broccoli
Cranberries	Brussels sprouts
Grapes	Cabbage
Kiwifruit	Carrots
Mango	Cauliflower
Oranges	Corn
Peaches	Kale
Pears	Onions
Plums	Radishes
Pomegranates	Romaine lettuce
Prunes	Spinach
Raisins	Sweet potatoes
Raspberries	Swiss chard
Strawberries	Turnip greens
Tomatoes	Winter squash

GOOD SOURCES OF OMEGA-3 FATS

- **Fish and seafood:** Anchovies, cod, crab, herring, lobster, mackerel, salmon, sardines, scallops, trout, tuna
- **Beans:** Kidney, mung, pinto
- **Nuts and seeds:** Flaxseed, pecans, pine nuts, walnuts
- **Oils:** Canola, flaxseed, cod liver, soybean

SMART SNACK COMBINATIONS

- Walnuts and raisins
- Celery sticks with natural almond butter
- Sliced apple with string cheese
- Yogurt mixed with blueberries
- Sardines on whole-grain crackers

SUPPLEMENTS USED FOR MEMORY AND BRAIN HEALTH

- **Anti-inflammatory supplements.** Omega-3 fatty acids (fish oil), curcumin
- **Antioxidants.** Vitamin E, acetyl-L-carnitine, coenzyme Q10, ginkgo biloba
- **B vitamins.** Folate (vitamin B9), cobalamin (vitamin B12)
- **Vitamin D**

- Melatonin
- Phosphatidylserine
- Huperzine A
- Apoaequorin

DO CHOLESTEROL DRUGS HELP MEMORY?

In general, taking a statin cholesterol-lowering drug is good for the brain. A number of investigations including thousands of volunteers aged seventy-five and older indicate that taking statins does bolster brain health and lower the risk for Alzheimer's disease. However, if someone already has Alzheimer's dementia, treatment with a statin drug has no better effect than taking a placebo. In a small number of people, statin medicines can cause memory loss or confusion as a side effect. Fortunately, when these patients stop taking the medicine, their memory improves.

DRUGS FOR TREATING ALZHEIMER'S SYMPTOMS

- **Aricept (donepezil).** Given orally for mild, moderate, or severe dementia
- **Exelon (rivastigmine).** Often given as a transdermal patch for mild or moderate dementia or dementia associated with Parkinson's disease

- **Namenda (memantine).** Given orally for moderate or severe dementia and often combined with either Aricept or Exelon
- **Namzaric.** A single pill that combines donepezil and memantine
- **Razadyne (galantamine).** Another anticholinergic medicine given orally for mild to moderate dementia

ADDITIONAL RESOURCES

There is no shortage of resources geared toward the elderly population, especially as medicine and science continue to make groundbreaking discoveries in the areas of aging and brain research and baby boomers mature into retirement at a rate of thousands per day. Consult the resources below in order to get yourself or a loved one on the road to healthful aging.

NAME	DESCRIPTION	TELEPHONE
AARP 601 E Street NW Washington, DC 20049 www.aarp.org	Nonprofit that helps older Americans achieve independence, dignity, and purpose	888-687-2277
Administration for Community Living 330 C St SW Washington, DC 20201 www.acl.gov	Provides information for older Americans and their families to enrich their lives and support their independence	202-401-4634
Alzheimer Europe 14, rue Dicks L-1417 Luxembourg www.alzheimer-europe.org	Organizes caregiver support and raises awareness about dementia in Europe	352-29-79-70

NAME	DESCRIPTION	TELEPHONE
Alzheimer's Association 225 N. Michigan Avenue, Fl. 17 Chicago, IL 60601 www.alz.org	Provides information on services, programs, publications, and local chapters	800-272-3900
Alzheimer's Foundation of America 322 Eighth Avenue, 16th floor New York, NY 10001 www.alzfdn.org	Supports organizations that improve quality of life of Alzheimer's patients and their caregivers	866-232-8484
Alzheimer's Disease Education & Referral Center PO Box 8250 Silver Spring, MD 20907 www.alzheimers.gov	National Institute on Aging service that distributes information on topics relevant to professionals, patients and their families, and the general public	800-438-4380
American Academy of Neurology 201 Chicago Avenue Minneapolis, MN 55415 www.aan.com	Professional organization that advances the art and science of neurology and promotes the best possible care for patients with neurological disorders	800-879-1960
American Association for Geriatric Psychiatry 6728 Old McLean Village Drive McLean, VA 22101 www.aagponline.org	Professional organization dedicated to enhancing the mental health and well-being of older adults through education and research	703-718-6026 703-556-9222

NAME	DESCRIPTION	TELEPHONE
American Geriatrics Society 40 Fulton Street, Suite 809 New York, NY 10038 www.americangeriatrics.org	Professional association providing assistance in identifying local geriatric physician referrals	212-308-1414 800-247-4779
American Psychiatric Association 800 Main Avenue, S.W., Suite 900 Washington, DC 20024 www.psych.org	Medical specialty society that works to ensure humane care and effective treatment for people with mental disorders	888-357-7924 202-559-3900
American Psychological Association 750 First Street NE Washington, DC 20002-4242 www.apa.org	Professional organization that represents US psychology and promotes health, education, and human welfare	800-374-2721 202-336-5500
American Society on Aging 548 Market Street, PMB 85589 San Francisco CA, 94104-5401 www.asaging.org	National organization concerned with physical, emotional, social, economic, and spiritual aspects of aging	415-974-9600 800-537-9728
ClinicalTrials.gov www.clinicaltrials.gov	Registry of federal and private clinical trials with information on contacts, locations, and trial purposes	

NAME	DESCRIPTION	TELEPHONE
Dana Alliance for Brain Initiatives 1270 Avenue of the Americas, 12th floor New York, NY 10020 www.dana.org	Organization that advances public awareness about the progress and benefits of brain research	212-223-4040
Gerontological Society of America 1220 L Street NW, Suite 901 Washington, DC 20005 www.geron.org	National interdisciplinary organization on research and education in aging	202-842-1275
The Healthy Brain Initiative www.cdc.gov/aging/healthybrain/index.htm	A road map from the CDC and Alzheimer's Association to advance cognitive health as a vital, integral component of public health	
Monterey Bay Aquarium Seafood Watch www.seafoodwatch.org	Comparison of the mercury levels of different fish	
National Center for Complementary and Integrative Health 31 Center Drive, MSC 2182 Building 31, Room 2B-11 Bethesda, MD 20892-2182 www.nccih.nih.gov	The branch of the National Institutes of Health dedicated to exploring complementary and alternative healing practices in the context of rigorous science	888-644-6226

NAME	DESCRIPTION	TELEPHONE
National Council on Aging 251 18th Street South, Suite 500 Arlington, VA 22202 www.ncoa.org	A network of organizations and individuals dedicated to improving the health and independence of older persons and increasing their continuing contributions to society	571-527-3900
National Institute of Mental Health 6001 Executive Boulevard, Room 6200, MSC 9663 Bethesda, MD 20892 www.nimh.nih.gov	The branch of the National Institutes of Health that focuses on biomedical and behavioral research	866-615-6464
National Institute of Neurological Disorders and Stroke PO Box 5801 Bethesda, MD 20824 www.ninds.nih.gov	The National Institutes of Health agency that supports neuroscience research; focuses on translating discoveries into prevention, treatment, and cures; and provides resource support and information	800-352-9424
National Institute on Aging Building 31, Room 5C27 31 Center Drive, MSC 2292 Bethesda, MD 20892-2292 www.nia.nih.gov/	One of the 27 institutes and centers of the National Institutes of Health; primary federal agency supporting and conducting Alzheimer's disease research	800-222-2225

NAME	DESCRIPTION	TELEPHONE
SeniorNet 6701 Koll Center Parkway, Suite 250 Pleasanton, CA 94566 www.seniornet.org	National nonprofit organization that works to build a community of computer-using seniors	239-275-2202
UCLA Longevity Center 760 Westwood Plaza, Room 38-261 Los Angeles, CA 90095-6980 www.semel.ucla.edu/longevity	University center that works to enhance and extend productive and healthy life through research and education on aging	310-794-0676
US Dept. of Veterans Affairs 810 Vermont Avenue NW Washington, DC 20420 www.va.gov	Provides information on VA programs, veterans benefits, VA facilities worldwide, and VA medical automation software	800-698-2411

LOWER YOUR ODDS FOR DEMENTIA WITH FOODS THAT FIGHT INFLAMMATION

Eating lots of fruits, veggies, beans and other foods with inflammation-cooling properties may lower your odds of developing dementia as you age.

But, if your diet is loaded with pro-inflammatory foods, you may be up to three times more likely to experience memory loss and issues with language, problem-solving and other thinking skills as you age, new research suggests.

"A less inflammatory diet relates to less risk for developing dementia," said study author Dr. Nikolaos Scarmeas, an associate professor of neurology at National and Kapodistrian University of Athens in Greece.

Exactly how, or even if, diet can help stave off dementia and preserve brain health isn't fully understood yet. "Diet may affect brain health via many mechanisms, and according to our findings, inflammation may be one of them," Scarmeas said.

For the study, more than 1,000 people in Greece (average age: 73) completed a questionnaire to determine the inflammatory potential or score of their diet. No one had dementia when the study began. Six percent developed dementia during a follow-up of just over three years.

Dietary inflammation scores range from -8.87 to 7.98, with higher scores pointing to a more inflammatory diet. Folks with the lowest scores were less likely to develop dementia than folks with higher ones, the study showed.

Each 1-point increase in dietary inflammatory score was associated with a 21% increase in dementia risk.

Those with the lowest scores consumed about 20 servings of fruit, 19 of vegetables, 4 of beans or other legumes, and 11 of coffee or tea each week. In contrast, people with the highest scores ate about 9 servings of fruit, 10 of vegetables, 2 of legumes, and 9 of coffee or tea per week.

It's not the whole food per se, but all the nutrients it contains that contributes to its inflammatory potential, Scarmeas explained. Each food has both pro- and anti-inflammatory ingredients.

"In general, a diet with more fruits, vegetables, beans, tea or coffee is a more anti-inflammatory one," he said.

The study does not prove that eating an anti-inflammatory diet prevents brain aging and dementia, only that there's a link between them.

Longer follow-up is needed to draw any firm conclusions on how inflammatory diet score affects brain health, Scarmeas cautioned.

The findings were published Nov. 10 in the journal *Neurology*.

Dr. Thomas Holland, a physician-scientist at Rush University Medical Center in Chicago, reviewed the findings.

"This study is lending further weight to the mechanism inflammation—specifically neuro-inflammation—that much of us understand as being one of the main players in causing cognitive decline and Alzheimer's dementia," he said.

Alzheimer's disease is the most common form of dementia.

For brain health, Holland recommends the MIND diet, the Mediterranean diet or the DASH diet. All three center on lean meats, fish, whole grains, fresh produce and olive oil. The MIND (or Mediterranean-DASH Intervention for Neurodegenerative Delay) diet combines elements from the Mediterranean and DASH diets and was specifically designed to help combat dementia.

So what should you eat to help boost brain health? Holland offered his suggestions.

"Berries, dark leafy greens, nuts, whole wheat, garlic, onions, peppers, tomatoes, extra virgin olive oil, non-fried dark fish, and poultry," he said.

These foods may decrease the strength and/or duration of the inflammatory process in your body and brain, Holland said. Some act as antioxidants, which sop up damaging free radicals and lower inflammation.

"Avoiding a Western-type diet pattern is also important, including reduced intake of whole-fat dairy, fried or fast foods, pastries and red meat," he said.

Holland noted that pro-inflammatory foods can lead to uncontrolled inflammation and damage.

"If that damage occurs in the brain, the potential to develop dementia exists," he said.

SOURCES: Nikolaos Scarmeas, MD, associate professor, neurology, National and Kapodistrian University of Athens, Greece; Thomas Holland, MD, MS, physician-scientist, Rush University, Chicago; *Neurology*, Nov. 10, 2021

THIS TWO-MINUTE MORNING ACTIVITY WILL BOOST YOUR ENERGY AND FOCUS ALL DAY

While a cup of coffee can start your morning with a bang, there's an easy, two-minute activity that will jumpstart your metabolism and give you more energy throughout the day. Uber investor Sahil Bloom developed the 5-5-5-30 morning exercise routine that takes only two minutes and has been scientifically shown to improve your attention, concentration, and learning and memory functions for the next two hours. You can do it while your coffee is brewing! And experts say that even two minutes of vigorous activity daily can boost your health as well.

According to Inc.com, Bloom's two-minute, full-body workout doesn't put significant stress on any one body part. Here's the breakdown:

- 5 pushups
- 5 squats

- 5 lunges
- and hold a 30-second plank

These five exercises can improve mental health and cognitive function, according to a meta-analysis published in *Transitional Sports Medicine*, that found only two minutes of effort yields two hours of focus and productivity.

In order to reap the rewards of this two-minute program, make it a daily habit, say experts. Forming new habits can enhance your fitness in 2023, and Bloom's 5-5-5-30 plan is just a suggestion. You can personalize the plan to include jumping jacks, walking up and down stairs or doing kettlebell swings for two minutes. Just choose exercises that involve the whole body.

Make sure that you do your two minutes first thing in the morning. One way to ensure success is to stack your habits, says Inc.com. For example, if you brush your teeth first thing upon rising, brush your teeth AFTER you exercise. If you are the kind of person who can't stand the thought of doing anything before you've had that first cup of coffee, that's the perfect habit to link with a two-minute workout. Make it a rule that you'll always do the 5-5-5-30 workout before you take the first sip.

You'll have a double dose of energy from your workout and the cup of java to start your day. Not only will you feel better, you'll be lowering your risk of developing several long-term conditions, such as cancer and heart disease, according to research published in the European Heart Journal.

Two-minute bursts of vigorous physical activity—totaling 15 minutes a week—are associated with a reduced risk of early death. The researchers defined vigorous activity as an increase in heart rate where people will often need to pause for breath when speaking, according to *Medical News Today*. Examples of vigorous physical activity include sprints, high intensity interval training (HIIT), swimming, or cycling at fast speed.

For the study, 71,893 men and women with no evidence of cardiovascular disease or cancer were selected from the U.K. Biobank study, a prospective cohort of people between ages 40 and 69. The participants who did no physical activity had a 4% risk of dying within five years. This risk was slashed in half with less than 10 minutes of daily vigorous physical activity and was halved again to a 1% risk if people did 60 minutes or more daily, says Medical News Today.

"This may be particularly important for people who do not have the time or do not wish to go to a gym or engage in 'traditional exercise'," said lead author Matthew Ahmadi, a postdoctoral research fellow at the University of Sydney in Australia. "We found as little as 15 minutes of vigorous physical activity per week can lower all-cause mortality and cancer risk by 15%, and 20 minutes per week can lower heart disease risk by 40%, with additional health benefits up to approximately 50 to 60 minutes per week."

ABOUT THE AUTHORS

GARY SMALL, M.D., and **GIGI VORGAN** are the authors of the *New York Times* bestseller *The Memory Bible*, as well as *The Memory Prescription*, *The Longevity Bible*, *iBrain*, *The Other Side of the Couch*, *The Alzheimer's Prevention Program*, *2 Weeks to a Younger Brain*, *SNAP! Change Your Personality in 30 Days*, *The Small Guide to Anxiety*, *The Small Guide to Alzheimer's Disease*, and *The Small Guide to Depression*. Dr. Small is chair of psychiatry at Hackensack University Medical Center and physician in chief for behavioral health at Hackensack Meridian Health, New Jersey's largest and most comprehensive health care network. Prior to joining Hackensack Meridian Health, Small was a professor of psychiatry and aging at the David Geffen School of Medicine at UCLA, director of the Division of Geriatric Psychiatry at the Semel Institute, and director of the UCLA Longevity Center. Named one of the world's top fifty innovators in science and technology by *Scientific American*, he has appeared frequently on *Today, Good Morning America*, PBS, and CNN and lectures throughout the world. In addition to working as coauthor with her husband Dr. Small, Ms. Vorgan has written feature films and television. She and Dr. Small live together in Weehawken, New Jersey.

For more information on their books and Dr. Small's appearances, visit DrGarySmall.com.

Notes

_____

_____

_____

_____

_____

_____

_____

_____

_____

_____

_____

_____

_____

_____

_____